cut the fat!

cut the fat!

More than 500 Easy and Enjoyable Ways to Reduce Fat from Every Meal

The American Dietetic Association

HarperPerennial

A Division of HarperCollins Publishers

FIRST EDITION

Designed by Laura Lindgren

0-06-273391-5

96 97 98 99 00 ❖/OPM 10 9 8 7 6 5 4 3

Contents

Introduction

If you've picked up this book to browse through the wealth of fat-cutting tips, you probably have an interest in reducing the amount of fat in your diet. Perhaps you've been told that your health depends on lowering your blood cholesterol level or weight, or you might have read in magazines and newspapers about the benefits of eating less fat, or maybe you're just interested in improving your overall health and level of fitness. Whatever the reason, this book is a good starting point for anyone new to eating less fat, as well as for the experienced fat-cutter looking for new ideas.

WHAT'S IN IT FOR ME?

Regardless of your current health and weight, eating low-fat provides short- and long-term benefits to people of all ages. A low-fat eating pattern can help you:

1. Reduce your risk for heart disease. Eating patterns that are high in fat, especially saturated fat, tend to raise blood cholesterol levels and increase the risk of heart disease and stroke. If you smoke, if you're carrying extra weight around your belly, if you have high blood pressure, or if you have a family history of heart disease, your risk is even greater.

2. Lower your odds of developing cancer. Diets that are high in fat are associated with certain types of cancer, including breast and colon cancer.

3. Decrease your body weight. Because fat is a concentrated source of calories, making even small changes in your eating style can add up to big savings over time. For example, if for the next year you reduced your usual fat intake by approximately 10 grams a day, you could expect to lose about 10 pounds! Add regular physical activity to the equation and you could enjoy other health benefits, including loss of body fat and increased energy. If you have high blood pressure, diabetes, or arthritis, you may even enjoy relief from your symptoms.

4. Feel better! As you lower the amount of fat you eat, you'll have room to enjoy more energy- and nutrient-packed foods, like fruits, vegetables, and grains.

THE FACTS ON FAT

Although fat has been given a bad name with many people needing to reduce their fat intake, it is an essential part of your diet. Fat provides the body with a major source of energy, carries and stores fat-soluble vitamins (vitamins A, D, E, and K), and also cushions and protects vital organs. In food it serves a number of purposes—blending and softening flavors, contributing to texture and color, and helping to provide a feeling of satisfaction after eating.

The challenge of eating less fat lies in learning how much is enough. To keep your fat intake below the recommended 30% or less of total calories from fat, use the following figures as a rough estimate of your daily fat allowance:

If you eat this many calories:	Allow yourself up to this much fat:
1200	40 grams
1400	47 grams
1600	53 grams
1800	60 grams
2000	65 grams
2200	73 grams
2400	80 grams
2800	93 grams

Do you wonder how many calories you should be consuming?

◆ 1600 calories is about right for many sedentary women and some older adults.

◆ 2200 calories is about right for most children, teenage girls, active women, and sedentary men. Women who are pregnant or breast-feeding will need somewhat more.

- 2800 calories is about right for teenage boys, many active men, and some very active women.

Use the Food Guide Pyramid and information on page 14 to help determine the amount of food that matches each calorie level.

SOME BASICS ON FAT AND CHOLESTEROL

Fat is found in many foods derived from both plants and animals. It is made up of three subtypes of fat. You'll often see these fats listed on the Nutrition Facts panel on most packaged foods.

- *Saturated fat* is found in large proportions in animal-based foods, including whole milk, cream, cheese, butter, meat, and poultry. It is also found in some plant-based foods, including coconut, palm, and palm kernel oils, and in hydrogenated oils. Saturated fat is generally more solid than other types of fats at room temperature.

◆ *Monounsaturated fat* is found in foods from both plants and animals. Olive, canola, and peanut oil all have large proportions of monounsaturated fat.

◆ *Polyunsaturated fat* is found in large proportions in many foods from plants, including sunflower, corn, soybean, cottonseed, and safflower oils. It is generally liquid at room temperature. Some varieties of fish are also sources of polyunsaturated fat, especially a type known as omega-3 fatty acids.

Other definitions you should know:

◆ *Cholesterol* is a waxy, fat-like substance produced in the bodies of all animals, including humans. Your body makes all the cholesterol it needs. All foods from animals—meat, poultry, fish, milk and milk products, and egg yolks—contain varying amounts of cholesterol. You can't see cholesterol in food. For example, both the lean and fat parts of meat and poultry contain cholesterol. Cholesterol is never found in foods from plants, even if they contain fat.

♦ *Hydrogenation* is a process that produces a more solid fat from an unsaturated liquid oil. It causes some of the unsaturated oil to become saturated and more solid. For example, a vegetable oil consisting primarily of polyunsaturated fat can be hydrogenated to a solid spreadable fat—margarine. During the hydrogenation process, some of the fats are changed to trans fatty acids. The term "trans" simply describes the chemical structure. Trans fatty acids are found in products containing hydrogenated oils and also occur naturally in beef, pork, lamb, butter, and milk. While there has been speculation of a potential link between trans fatty acids and increases in blood cholesterol levels, there is little scientific evidence to suggest that cutting back on your intake of certain foods only because of trans fatty acids is necessary.

By now you're probably wondering, "What type of fat should I be consuming?" Here's the bottom line—monounsaturated and polyunsaturated fats may help lower blood cholesterol levels when they *replace* saturated fat in the diet. However, this does not give you free reign to overindulge in these fats because cutting back on the *total* amount of fat *you consume* is most important.

PUTTING FAT AND CALORIES INTO PERSPECTIVE

Many foods contribute fat to your diet. Fat is a concentrated source of calories, providing more than twice as many calories as equivalent amounts of carbohydrate or protein. Because some foods contain more fat than others, you may have heard that lower-fat foods are *good* while higher-fat foods are *bad* and should be never be eaten. This notion is not only false, but also unwise. In addition to the pleasure of a great meal, all foods provide us with energy and essential nutrients. If you eliminated certain foods, your overall eating pattern would likely be missing essential nutrients obtained from consuming a variety of foods. More importantly, you might lose some of the enjoyment of eating. Placing a value judgment on individual foods should be reserved for your individual taste buds!

Today we can delight in the wide selection of low-fat and fat-free products. While they offer excellent options for reducing the fat in your diet, these products still contain calories—sometimes even more calories than the full-fat product. If you're trying to control your weight, this is an important point to remember. If you don't care for the taste of some fat-modified products, you may find it more satisfying to eat a smaller amount—or have just one or two bites of a higher-fat food—than to substitute a low-fat or fat-free product. Use the tactic that works best for you.

You may have heard that a healthful diet should include no more than 30 percent of total calories from fat. The key message here is that your *overall diet*—not individual foods—should comply with this guideline. If you selected individual foods on the basis of this "30 percent rule," you would eliminate many delicious and nutritious foods, such as cheese, peanut butter, hamburgers, and most desserts. If you instead balance higher-fat foods with those lower in fat throughout the day and learn to make trade-offs, you can eat and enjoy any food!

MAKING TRADE-OFFS

Are some of your favorite foods high in fat? If so, you don't need to give these foods up—just trade them off! Should variety, balance, and moderation already characterize your eating style, use trade-offs to include some of your favorite high-fat foods in your diet.

Trading off is a simple strategy for keeping balance and moderation in your eating style. Balancing foods with less fat (or sugar or salt) with foods that have more—while keeping within nutrient and Food Guide Pyramid guidelines for good health—is its goal. With trade-offs, any food can fit in a healthful diet, including food with more fat. For example, choose a sandwich with low-fat cheese for lunch so you can spend the fat savings on a cookie for dessert. Refer to the tips in this guide to trade off and balance foods to lower your fat intake.

THE FOOD GUIDE PYRAMID

The Food Guide Pyramid is a practical tool that makes it easier to follow a low-fat eating style. Every food you eat fits into one or more of the food groups in the Pyramid.

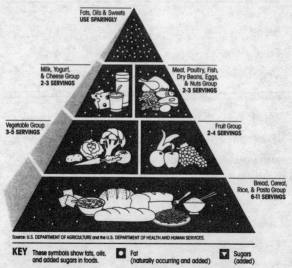

Fats, Oils & Sweets
USE SPARINGLY

Milk, Yogurt, & Cheese Group
2-3 SERVINGS

Meat, Poultry, Fish, Dry Beans, Eggs, & Nuts Group
2-3 SERVINGS

Vegetable Group
3-5 SERVINGS

Fruit Group
2-4 SERVINGS

Bread, Cereal, Rice, & Pasta Group
6-11 SERVINGS

Source: U.S. DEPARTMENT OF AGRICULTURE and the U.S. DEPARTMENT OF HEALTH AND HUMAN SERVICES.

KEY These symbols show fats, oils, and added sugars in foods. ● Fat (naturally occurring and added) ▼ Sugars (added)

♦ 13 ♦

The actual number of servings you need depends on your energy needs, which is determined by your age, sex, body size, and activity level. Pages 5–6 explained how many calories you need based on the above criteria. Here are suggestions for how many servings you should be choosing from each food group:

Food Group	1600 Calories	2200 Calories	2800 Calories
Bread	6	9	11
Fruit	2	3	4
Vegetable	3	4	5
Milk	2–3[1]	2–3[1]	2–3[1]
Meat	5 ounces	6 ounces	7 ounces

[1]*Pregnant and breast-feeding women, teenagers, and young adults to age twenty-four need three servings.*

What Is a Serving?

Using moderation as a guiding principle of healthful eating means choosing *reasonable* portions of foods. While you may not always consume a "standard" serving, keep the recommended serving sizes in mind as you plan your meals and tally your food choices from each food group. You don't need to measure every serving, just use this information as a general guide.

- Bread, Cereal, Rice, and Pasta
  1 slice of bread, ½ bagel, ½ hamburger or hot dog bun, ½ English muffin
  1 ounce of ready-to-eat cereal (check the Nutrition Facts panel for the cup measure)
  ½ cup of oatmeal or other cooked cereal, ½ cup of cooked rice or pasta

- Vegetables
  1 cup of raw leafy vegetables, such as spinach
  ½ cup of other vegetables, cooked or chopped raw (like cauliflower, brussels sprouts, asparagus)
  ¾ cup of vegetable juice

- Fruits
  1 medium apple, banana, orange, kiwi, pear, peach, nectarine, tangerine
  ½ cup of canned, freshly-chopped, or cooked fruit, such as mandarin oranges, peach halves, melon, berries, grapes, prunes
  ¾ cup of fruit juice

- Milk, Yogurt, and Cheese
  1 cup of milk or yogurt
  1½ ounces of natural cheese, 2 ounces of processed cheese

- Meat, Poultry, Seafood, Dry Beans, Eggs, and Nuts
  2–3 ounces of cooked lean meat, poultry, or fish
  ½ cup of cooked dry beans, 1 egg, or 2 tablespoons of peanut butter count as 1 ounce of meat

THE FOOD LABEL

Food labels provide valuable information about the foods you eat and can help you make wise choices at the supermarket. Regarding fat content information, the Nutrition Facts panel on most packaged food includes the number of grams of total fat and saturated fat and the number of milligrams of cholesterol per serving of food.

The Percent Daily Value (% Daily Value) on the food label is a yardstick to measure the amount of certain nutrients contained in a serving of food against your overall needs. For example, if a food contains 13 grams (g) of fat, is this a lot or a little? To find out, use the information in the % Daily Value column. You'll see that 13 grams is 20% of your daily allowance of fat (65 grams), based on a 2000 calorie diet. The Percent Daily Value helps make sense of the nutrition numbers on the label by putting the amount of fat found in a serving of the food in the context of your total diet.

You can also use the words on the front of the food label to find foods with less total fat, saturated fat, and cholesterol.

If the Label Says:	It Means:
Fat Free	Less than 0.5 g fat per serving
Low Fat	3 g or less fat per serving
Reduced Fat, Less Fat	At least 25% less fat per serving when compared with a similar food
Saturated Fat Free	Less than 0.5 g saturated fat per serving
Low Saturated Fat	1 g or less saturated fat per serving and no more than 15% of calories from saturated fat
Reduced or Less Saturated Fat	At least 25% less saturated fat per serving when compared with a similar food
Cholesterol Free	Less than 2 mg cholesterol per serving and 2 g or less saturated fat per serving
Low Cholesterol	20 mg or less cholesterol per serving and 2 g or less saturated fat per serving

Lean	Packaged seafood or game meat, cooked meat, or cooked poultry with less than 10 g total fat, less than 4 g saturated fat, and less than 95 mg cholesterol per serving
Extra Lean	Packaged seafood or game meat, cooked meat, or cooked poultry with less than 5 g total fat, less than 2 g saturated fat, and less than 95 mg cholesterol per serving
Light or Lite	At least ⅓ fewer calories or 50% less fat per serving; if more than half the calories are from fat, fat content must be reduced by 50% or more. Nonnutrient "light" or "lite" claims are allowed, but must identify the basis for the claim. *Examples*: "light in color," "light in texture."

WHERE DO I BEGIN?

Cut the Fat! provides simple ideas for reducing the amount of fat you eat in various situations and settings—whether you're at home experiencing a snack attack, at a Mexican restaurant, on an airplane, or at a cookout. Anytime and anywhere, just flip to the corresponding section to find some easy-to-use fat-reducing tips. Besides hundreds of suggestions for choosing and preparing foods with less fat, *Cut the Fat!* also provides some fun facts and quick, tasty, and easy-to-prepare low-fat recipes. Don't be surprised if you end up loving low-fat eating!

Cut the Fat! has yet another great feature—its size. It's small enough to carry with you wherever you go. You'll always have a fat-fighting resource at your fingertips. Take it slow and, even though it may be tempting, don't try to make all the changes at once. Pick a couple of tips to work on, and once you've mastered these, try some others. Different days, situations, and locations will require different strategies, so always be prepared to try some new fat-cutting techniques.

Remember, small changes can add up to big fat savings. Once you discover the wonderful taste of a low-fat eating style, you'll never want to go back!

At the Grocery Store

Preparing lower-fat foods to eat at home and "on the go" depends on what you bring home from the grocery store. Shop with a list to help limit the number of high-fat foods you purchase on a whim. And shop after you've eaten so you're not tempted to buy too many high-fat snacks and desserts to satisfy your growling stomach.

BREAD, CEREAL, RICE, AND PASTA

Buy whole-grain breads for a low-fat, high-fiber source of complex carbohydrates, B vitamins, and iron—look for breads with whole-wheat flour, stone-ground whole-wheat flour, or 100 percent whole-wheat flour listed first on the ingredient listing.

◆

Sourdough, white, oatmeal, and Italian and French breads are also low in fat or fat-free.

◆

Add variety as you choose low-fat breads —try bagels, English muffins, and pita bread.

◆

Buy soft corn or flour tortillas for tacos, Mexican pizzas, or salads. The soft varieties contain less fat than the fried, crispy versions, and soft corn tortillas generally have less fat than soft flour tortillas. Fat-free tortillas may also be available in your supermarket.

◆

Fill your shopping cart with pasta, rice, and other grains like bulgur, quinoa, and barley. These are naturally low in fat and are good sources of complex carbohydrates and fiber.

◆

Packaged rice and pasta dishes are often high in fat. Decrease the fat by eliminating or cutting back on the amount of oil or margarine called for in the package directions.

◆

Save about 1.5 grams of fat per 1-cup serving by purchasing yolkless noodles rather than egg noodles.

◆

Ready-to-eat cereals are generally low in fat, with the exception of some granola cereals. If you like granola, look for low-fat varieties.

◆

Potato and tortilla chips are available in baked versions, which usually contain less than 1 gram of fat per serving. Look for naturally low-fat salsas or reduced-fat dips to accompany these.

◆

Rice cakes, popcorn cakes, and pretzels are low-fat or fat-free snack options.

◆

Naturally low-fat cracker options include saltines, rye crackers, crispbreads, melba toasts and rounds, zwieback, and bread sticks.

◆

Look for reduced-fat versions of your favorite snack crackers. You can save 2 to 3 grams of fat per serving.

◆

Many traditional cookie favorites are naturally low in fat, including fig and other fruit bars, gingersnaps, graham crackers, vanilla wafers, and animal crackers.

◆

Look for reduced-fat or fat-free versions of other cookie favorites. You can save about 2 grams of fat per serving.

◆

Buy reduced-fat cake mixes or angel food cake mixes for low-fat desserts and top with fresh fruit or a fat-free glaze (see recipe in *At Home: Desserts* section, page 100) instead of frosting.

◆

Look for dry bread crumbs and croutons without added fat or make your own.

FRUITS AND VEGETABLES

Fruits and vegetables are packed with vitamins, minerals, and fiber, and most are fat-free—avocados and olives are the exceptions.

> Choose a variety of dark-green, orange, and yellow fruits and vegetables. Broccoli, carrots, spinach, chard, sweet potatoes, apricots, mangoes, cantaloupes, and peaches are all excellent sources of vitamin A (beta-carotene). Combined with a low-fat diet, these may help lower your risk for some types of cancer. The vitamin C in fruits and vegetables may also help reduce the risk of certain cancers. Good sources include citrus fruits, strawberries, kiwis, tomatoes, and peppers.

◆

Fill up on fiber-containing fruits and vegetables and you won't have as much room for higher-fat foods.

◆

Stock up on fresh fruit—use these as quick snacks and desserts.

◆

Buy canned or frozen vegetables without butter, cream, or cheese sauces and enjoy the flavor of the vegetable itself with a sprinkle of lemon juice, imitation butter flakes, or your favorite seasoning.

◆

Better yet, buy fresh vegetables. Eat them raw for crunchy snacks, or steam or stir-fry for full-flavor accompaniments to meals.

◆

Dried fruits such as raisins, prunes, apricots, and dates are fat-free, easy to store and transport, and delicious alternatives to fresh fruits.

◆

To be sure that you always have fruits and vegetables on hand, keep a stock of canned varieties in your cupboard and bags of frozen vegetables and fruits in your freezer.

◆

Look for broth-based soups with lots of legumes and other vegetables—these contain considerably less fat than cream-based soups. Or buy reduced-fat varieties of cream-based soups and add frozen or canned vegetables to boost the flavor while adding vitamins and minerals.

◆

If you live alone, remember that individual portions of naturally low-fat fresh fruits and vegetables are available at your local grocery or deli salad bar. Select just enough of your favorites to last one or two days.

◆

Precut, packaged vegetables in the produce section make quick side dishes and salads for low-fat meals.

MEAT, POULTRY, SEAFOOD, DRY BEANS, EGGS, AND NUTS

For a quick meal, try one of the many frozen entrées that are low-fat and portioned in single-serving sizes.

◆

Choose cuts of beef with the words "loin" or "round" in the name. These contain as little as 3 grams of fat per 3-ounce cooked and trimmed portion.

◆

Check the grade of beef also—"Choice" and "Select" grades have less marbling and contribute the least amount of fat.

◆

Look for meats with all visible fat trimmed. There's an average of 42% less fat in trimmed cuts than untrimmed cuts.

◆

Choose ground beef with the highest percent lean on the label or look for packages with the words "loin" or "round" in the name, such as ground sirloin and ground round.

◆

When buying pork, look for cuts with the word "loin" in the name. These contain as little as 4 grams of fat per 3-ounce cooked and trimmed portion.

◆

Lower-fat veal cuts are veal arm or blade steak, rib roast, loin chops, and veal cutlets. These contain 5 to 6 grams of fat per 3-ounce cooked and trimmed portion.

◆

When choosing lamb, look for the following cuts, which contain 5 to 8 grams of fat per 3-ounce cooked and trimmed portion: arm chop, shank, loin chop, and leg roast.

◆

White meat chicken and turkey, such as the breast and wing portions, have an average of 5 grams of fat less per 3-ounce serving than dark meat (thigh and drumstick).

◆

For convenience and less fat, buy boneless, skinless breasts of chicken or turkey. Or buy poultry with the skin on and remove it before eating to save up to 5 grams of fat per 3-ounce serving.

◆

For ground turkey with the least amount of fat, look for the words "ground skinless turkey meat" on the label or ask your butcher to grind breast meat without the skin.

◆

When buying whole turkey, be aware that "self-basting" varieties are high in fat. Look for a turkey without that label; keep it moist by frequently basting it yourself with broth, juice, or the natural juices from the bird. Also, roasting the bird with the breast side up maintains moistness.

◆

Most chicken and turkey nuggets, patties, and rolls include ground skin. Look for products made with whole chicken or turkey pieces or strips—preferably light meat—for less fat.

◆

Choose white-meat fish, such as cod, flounder, sole, and orange roughy. These have less fat than darker-meat fish, like salmon, bluefin tuna, and mackerel.

◆

When buying luncheon meats, choose lean ham, beef, and turkey breast from the deli and have them sliced thinly. You'll probably use less meat on your sandwich and lower your fat intake as a result.

◆

Look at the labels on packaged lunch meats and choose varieties with the least fat per serving. Packaged meats that are up to 97% fat-free still contain fat, so be sure to read the labels closely. Fat-free luncheon meats are also available.

◆

Many varieties of lower-fat hot dogs are available. These generally contain less than 4 grams of fat per frank, compared with regular varieties at 11 to 13 grams per frank. Turkey and chicken franks do not always contain less fat than beef franks—some are just smaller. Fat-free hot dogs are also an option.

◆

Choose lean smoked ham, Canadian bacon, or low-fat turkey versions of bacon instead of regular bacon to save on fat without losing flavor.

◆

Egg substitutes can replace whole eggs in many recipes. Most contain only egg whites and no fat, while some are egg white / whole egg blends and contain 2 to 3 grams of fat per ½ cup. You'll find cartons of egg substitutes in the refrigerator and freezer cases of your grocery store.

♦

Most legumes (dried beans and peas), such as kidney beans, navy beans, lima beans, chickpeas, lentils, and split peas, are very low in fat and supply fiber, protein, folic acid, iron, and other minerals. For a time-saver, buy canned beans instead of dried.

♦

Look for lower-fat versions of peanut butter. These contain about 12 grams of fat per 2-tablespoon serving, compared with 17 grams per 2-tablespoon serving in regular varieties.

◆

Nuts, regardless of whether they are dry-roasted or oil-roasted, contain about the same amount of fat—ranging from 14 to 22 grams per ounce. Seeds such as sunflower and sesame are also concentrated fat sources. Buy seeds and nuts to use in small amounts as flavor enhancers for salads, breads, stir-fries, and vegetables.

MILK, YOGURT, AND CHEESE

Skim milk contains the least amount of fat per 1-cup serving (just a trace), compared with 2.6 grams in 1%, 4.7 grams in 2%, and 8.9 grams in whole milk.

◆

Even small amounts of half-and-half or whipping cream in coffee add up. Look for reduced-fat or light powdered nondairy creamers, which generally contain only 1 gram of fat per tablespoon.

◆

If chocolate milk is a favorite, look for 1% fat varieties or buy skim milk and add chocolate syrup or a chocolate powder mix.

◆

Yogurts come in many different varieties. Look for nonfat or low-fat products. Custard-style or whole-milk yogurts contain 6 to 8 grams of fat per 8-ounce serving, compared with about 0 to 4 grams of fat in nonfat and low-fat yogurts.

> To save about 3 grams of fat in a recipe calling for buttermilk, substitute "mock" buttermilk made by adding about 2 teaspoons of lemon juice or vinegar to each cup of skim milk. Let this mixture sit for 5 minutes before adding to the recipe.

Despite its name, buttermilk contains about 2 to 3 grams of fat per 1-cup serving—making it comparable to 1% milk. Another option is to add dry buttermilk, which contains about 0.5 gram of fat per tablespoon, to skim milk.

◆

Eggnog is available in low-fat versions. Look for the words "low-fat" or "1%" or "2% milkfat" on the label. While regular eggnog contains about 19 grams of fat per 1-cup serving, a 1% milkfat version contains only 4 grams of fat per cup.

◆

The amount of fat in cheeses varies by variety, as well as by whether or not it's reduced in fat. Most varieties, like cheddar, American, Swiss, Colby, blue, Gouda, feta, and Monterey Jack, contain 8 to 10 grams of fat per 1-ounce serving. (One ounce is equal to 1 slice or a chunk about the size of a thumb.) Compare these with reduced-fat or skim varieties, like part-skim mozzarella, which contain 2 to 6 grams of fat per 1-ounce serving. Try your favorite cheese in a low-fat or nonfat version—you might be surprised how similar they taste.

◆

Experiment with strong-flavored cheeses, like blue, Roquefort, Gorgonzola, and Gruyère. You may find that a small amount will add as much flavor to your foods—if not more—as a larger serving of a milder cheese.

◆

Buy hard cheeses like Parmesan and Romano in grated form or grate them yourself. One tablespoon contains under 2 grams of fat. Hard cheeses offer lots of flavor, so you can use less when you substitute them for shredded full-fat cheeses.

◆

Look for Neufchatel cheese or reduced-fat or nonfat cream cheeses. Neufchatel cheese is very similar in flavor to cream cheese. At 7 grams of fat per ounce, Neufchatel contains less fat than regular cream cheese containing 10 grams, but slightly more fat than reduced-fat versions with only 5 grams.

◆

Buy part-skim ricotta cheese at about 10 grams per ½-cup serving, compared with whole-milk ricotta at about 16 grams per ½-cup serving. Nonfat varieties are also available.

◆

Cottage cheese is available in fat-free (also called dry curd), 1% milkfat, and 4% milkfat varieties. Save about 7 grams of fat per cup by switching from 4% to 1% and save about 2 grams more by switching to a nonfat variety. There is no difference in fat content between the different curd sizes.

◆

In recipes that call for sour cream, you can reduce the fat by using low-fat or nonfat sour cream.

FATS, OILS, AND SWEETS

For everyday use, look for soft, tub margarines and spreads made with unsaturated oils. These varieties generally contain 11 to 12 grams of fat per tablespoon, so use them sparingly. Diet margarines, also referred to on labels as "light," "low-fat," or "reduced-calorie," contain more water and are whipped with air. These generally contain 6 or fewer grams of fat per tablespoon. Liquid margarines contain about 11 grams of fat per tablespoon.

◆

Butter in stick, spread, or tub form contains approximately the same amount of fat per tablespoon as margarine. The primary difference is that butter products contain cholesterol in addition to fat because butter is made from an animal product.

◆

Look for fruit butters, such as apple, apricot, peach, or pumpkin, to use as spreads on breads and crackers. Don't be fooled by the name—these are all fat-free!

Besides reading margarine labels for grams of fat per serving, also read the list of ingredients. Products with water or a liquid oil (one that is not hydrogenated or partially hydrogenated) listed as the first ingredients contain less saturated fat per serving. Types of oils to look for on margarine products include canola (rapeseed), safflower, and sunflower because these contain the smallest amounts of saturated fats. Since margarines are made from plant oils, no margarine products contain cholesterol.

♦

Buy mayonnaise, salad dressings, and sandwich spreads in light, low-fat/cholesterol-free, or fat-free varieties. Regular mayonnaise or salad dressing contains about 6 to 11 grams of fat per tablespoon, light products contain about 3 to 5 grams, and low-fat/cholesterol-free products contain about 1 gram.

♦

Oils are all very similar in the amount of fat—13 to 14 grams per tablespoon. Look for oils containing primarily unsaturated fats—these include olive, peanut, canola, safflower, sunflower, corn, and soybean oils.

◆

Choose stronger-flavored oils, such as extra virgin olive, hot chili, and sesame oil. Because of their stronger flavor, a smaller amount will go a long way in savory recipes and salads.

Wondering whether extra virgin, virgin, and light olive oil differ in the amount of fat? The difference is in the acid content, not the fat. Extra virgin olive oil comes from the first pressing of olives and is the most flavorful and usually the deepest color. New "light" olive oils are not lower in fat—the "light" refers to the lighter color, fragrance, and flavor.

◆

A can of vegetable oil spray is a handy fat-saver. Use this to prepare pans and casserole dishes for sautéing and baking to minimize the amount of fat added.

◆

Choose from the wide array of reduced-fat and fat-free salad dressings. Compared with regular oil- and cream-based salad dressings, which can contain up to 21 grams of fat per 2 tablespoons (often less than many people use!), reduced-fat and fat-free dressings usually contain 0 to 8 grams of fat per 2 tablespoons. Experiment until you find a brand and flavor you like.

◆

Try dry blends for mixing your own salad dressings and use less oil and more vinegar and water (or other flavorful liquids like juice or wine) than called for on the package directions.

◆

Ketchup, mustard, horseradish, chutney, salsas, and pickle relish are tasty, low-fat spreads. Use these products to boost flavor and reduce the amount of mayonnaise or salad dressing added to sandwiches and salads. They can also be used to complement the flavors of lean meat, poultry, and fish.

At Home

Your cupboards are stocked with low-fat foods and ingredients and your refrigerator and freezer are overflowing with fruits, vegetables, and low-fat dairy products and meats. You wonder how you'll combine these foods to make delicious and satisfying meals. Read on for easy ideas for eating low-fat at home.

BREAKFAST

Packaged waffle or pancake mixes make a quick, tasty breakfast. Look for those with no more than 5 grams of fat for a serving of 2 waffles or pancakes. Skip the 2 teaspoons of butter or margarine to save 8 grams of fat and use a fat-free topping, such as syrup, fresh fruit, jam or jelly, or fruit butter.

◆

Adjust your homemade French toast and pancake recipes to reduce the number of whole eggs used. Cook in a nonstick skillet coated with vegetable oil cooking spray instead of oil, butter, or margarine.

◆

For convenience, pop a frozen waffle or pancake in the toaster. Enjoy this instead of a glazed doughnut and save up to 12 grams of fat.

◆

Make a scrambled egg sandwich with toasted English muffins, a slice of Canadian bacon or lean ham, and a scrambled egg prepared in a nonstick skillet coated with vegetable oil cooking spray. To reduce fat even more, use ¼ cup of egg substitute or 2 egg whites instead of a whole egg to save 5 fat grams.

◆

For a low-fat, hot and spicy breakfast, make a quick breakfast burrito.

Breakfast Burrito

For each person, scramble 2 large egg whites or ¼ cup of egg substitute in a nonstick pan coated with vegetable oil cooking spray. While still hot, place on a small, warm corn or flour tortilla along with ¼ cup of low-fat or fat-free shredded cheddar cheese, roll up, and top with salsa.

◆

Prepare an omelet using 1 egg, 2 egg whites or ¼ cup of egg substitute, and a tablespoon of skim milk. Add vegetables (broccoli, mushrooms, onions); a tablespoon of shredded, sharp low-fat cheese; and seasonings—a pinch of oregano and black pepper—for extra flavor.

◆

Have a poached egg in place of your usual fried egg and save about 4 grams of fat.

◆

If you choose either 3 slices of bacon or 3 (½ ounce each) sausage links, you will add 9 to 12 grams of fat to your breakfast. Instead, try 3 slices of turkey bacon for 8 grams of fat or 3 slices of Canadian bacon for 6 grams of fat.

◆

Granola cereals tend to be higher in fat than others (though low-fat varieties are available). If you enjoy granola, try eating it three days a week and a low-fat or nonfat flake, shredded wheat, or oat cereal on the other days. Be sure to use skim or 1% milk.

◆

Replace the tablespoon of butter or margarine you usually spread on your toast, bagel, or English muffin with apple butter, jelly, or jam and save 11 to 12 grams of fat. Replace the ounce of cream cheese and save 10 grams of fat. For a change, try a crumpet (with or without tea) for a fat-free breakfast bread.

◆

Instead of a croissant, eat a bagel with fat-free cream cheese and save 10 grams of fat.

◆

Try a fruited bagel at about 1 gram of fat instead of a muffin and save at least 4 grams of fat.

◆

Make your own low-fat muffins using skim milk, egg whites or egg substitute, and equal parts fruit purée (prune or apricot), mashed bananas, or applesauce and oil to save on fat. Or buy a packaged mix and replace some or all of the added fat called for in the directions with fruit purée.

Fruit Purée

Combine 1⅓ cups (8 ounces) of pitted prunes or dried apricots with 6 tablespoons of hot water in a food processor and purée until smooth. Makes 1 cup. Can keep refrigerated for up to 2 months in a tightly sealed container.

◆

Purée nonfat or low-fat cottage cheese with chives, fresh fruit, or fruit preserves to spread on toast, bagels, waffles, or pancakes. Or make a yogurt spread.

Yogurt Spread

Place low-fat yogurt in a colander lined with cheesecloth or a double layer of white paper towels. Place the colander over a bowl to catch the draining liquid. Refrigerate overnight. Makes a smooth, thick spread you can use in place of cream cheese or sour cream in many recipes.

◆

For a low-fat breakfast on the go, grab a bagel or nonfat muffin, fresh fruit or juice box, and carton of low-fat or nonfat yogurt.

◆

For another quick breakfast or snack, blend until smooth ½ cup of nonfat yogurt, ½ cup of canned or 1 piece of fresh fruit, and 2 ice cubes. Add cinnamon or sugar to the desired sweetness.

◆

Use dried fruit (raisins, apricots, apples) or cinnamon, nutmeg, allspice, cloves, and ginger rather than butter or margarine to flavor hot, cooked cereals.

LUNCH AND DINNER

Sandwiches and Spreads

Rather than the usual tablespoon of mayonnaise on your sandwich, spread on a Dijon, honey, country style, tarragon, or other spicy mustard blend to save about 10 grams of fat. Horseradish alone or mixed with mustard adds a unique flavor to sandwiches. If a sandwich without mayonnaise just won't do, use a low-fat or fat-free variety.

◆

Other good spreads for sandwiches—as well as hamburgers and hot dogs—are ketchup, salsa, and barbecue or steak sauce, all of which are virtually fat-free.

◆

Salsa also makes a nice dip for fresh vegetables. It contains no fat, compared with 3 grams in just 1 ounce (a couple spoonfuls) of sour cream dip. Or use nonfat sour cream and mix in salsa for a dip with zip.

◆

Make a sandwich with about 3 ounces of sliced, skinless chicken or turkey, lean ham, or roast beef. Add a slice of low-fat or nonfat cheese and one of the low-fat or nonfat spreads mentioned above for a sandwich with less than 10 grams of fat.

◆

A ½ cup of tuna salad made with oil-packed light tuna and regular mayonnaise or salad dressing contains about 20 grams of fat. Using water-packed light tuna and low-fat or nonfat mayonnaise or salad dressing saves up to 18 grams of fat. Add some chopped vegetables and dried dill and pepper for flavor. Serve on whole-grain bread or a bagel, add a piece of fresh fruit and a glass of skim milk, and you have a balanced, low-fat lunch.

◆

Complement your sandwiches with crunchy, raw vegetable pieces like baby carrots, broccoli, or cucumbers instead of potato chips or french fries and save about 10 grams of fat.

cut the fat!

◆

Enjoy a low-fat hot dog with less than 4 grams of fat (at least 50% less fat than regular dogs). Or cut fat grams even further with fat-free hot dogs.

◆

Make a low-fat pizza topped with vegetables.

Pizza

Start with premade plain pizza shells or sliced French bread. Top with thin slices of your favorite vegetables, like tomato, zucchini, peppers, and mushrooms. Sprinkle with a tablespoon of grated hard cheese (Parmesan, Romano, Asiago) and seasonings like garlic, oregano, thyme, marjoram, or basil. Bake in a hot oven for 10 minutes.

◆

For pita sandwiches, try sautéed or steamed vegetables or turkey, lean ham, or roast beef with a low-fat dressing.

◆

Hummus with tomato, shredded lettuce, and a black olive or two also makes a tasty pita sandwich. Because some prepared hummus can be fairly high in fat, make your own lower-fat version.

Hummus

In a food processor, mince 2 cloves of garlic, add a 15-ounce can of chickpeas, rinsed and drained, the juice of a whole lemon, 3 table-spoons of tahini (sesame seed paste), and 1 to 2 teaspoons of paprika. Add water 2 tablespoons at a time until the desired consistency is reached. The hummus can be refrigerated in a closed container for up to one week. Sprinkle with additional paprika before serving. Serve with raw vegetables, pita bread, or baked pita chips.

Salads

Favorite pasta salads can be made using a fat-free Italian or other flavored dressing.

◆

Make a lower-fat antipasto salad by chopping or shredding the higher-fat ingredients and then using smaller amounts. For example, use diced olives, salami, and shredded part-skim mozzarella, then top with a fat-free Italian dressing.

◆

Reduce the fat in potato salad by using low-fat salad dressing or plain yogurt and reducing or eliminating the chopped hard-boiled eggs.

◆

For homemade salad dressings, replace some or all of the oil with water, vinegar, orange or lemon juice, dry or Dijon mustard, and a pinch of sugar or honey. Figure about 1 teaspoon of oil per person when making your own dressing. Experiment with flavored vinegars, such as balsamic, red wine, champagne, raspberry, or rice.

Salad Dressing

To create a salad dressing for four, shake together $\frac{1}{2}$ cup of red wine or rice vinegar, 4 teaspoons of peanut or olive oil, 1 tablespoon of honey or orange marmalade, and $\frac{1}{2}$ teaspoon of dried basil. Toss with salad greens.

◆

Replace high-fat soup or salad toppings, such as fried croutons, chow mein noodles, bacon bits, or sunflower seeds, with lower-fat crunchy options, like baked croutons, oyster crackers, celery chunks, or scallion slices.

◆

For fruit salad, use low-fat or nonfat yogurt and cinnamon as a topping.

◆

Make a taco or chef's salad in a baked tortilla bowl instead of a fried one and save up to 28 grams of fat.

Baked Tortilla Bowl

Place a round, oven-safe saucepan or dish (about 8 inches in diameter) on a cookie sheet. Spray with vegetable oil cooking spray. Gently push a 12-inch tortilla into the dish, forming a bowl. Spray the tortilla with cooking spray. To keep the bowl from collapsing during baking, place an oven-safe mug in the center. Bake at 450° for 10 to 12 minutes or until crisp. Fill with salad greens and vegetables, and top with low-fat dressing or plain yogurt mixed with fresh herbs.

◆

After washing your salad greens, dry them thoroughly with a salad spinner or paper towels. You'll use less salad dressing because it will coat the leafy greens instead of sliding off to the bottom of your salad bowl.

Soups, Chilies, and Stews

Broth, noodle, and vegetable soups are usually lowest in fat, with 2 to 3 grams per ½ cup. Most dry mixes are also low-fat. Look for those with pasta, vegetables, and legumes.

◆

When making cream-based soups, substitute skim or evaporated skim milk for the cream and add mashed potatoes or instant potato flakes for thickness and flavor.

◆

Add roasted red peppers or smoked turkey instead of ham hocks to homemade pea or bean soups or stews for smoky flavor without the fat.

◆

Use a slow-cooking pot to make a hearty stew with lean cubes of meat, vegetables, and tomato sauce. The long, slow, moist-heat cooking makes leaner, tougher cuts of meat juicy, tender, and flavorful.

◆

Substitute black, navy, or kidney beans for some or all of the ground meat in home-made chili.

◆

Place canned soups, broths, chilies, stews, or baked beans in the refrigerator for about 30 minutes before opening. Remove the lid and defat by skimming off the solidified fat. Some fat may also solidify and stick to the sides of the can. This method also works with homemade soups and stews. Just chill and then remove the fat that rises to the surface.

Meat, Poultry, and Seafood

Low-fat cooking methods for meat, poultry, and seafood include broiling, steaming, roasting, baking, microwaving, grilling, braising, boiling, poaching, and stir-frying (if a small amount of oil is used).

◆

Use nonstick cookware to reduce or eliminate the amount of fat needed for sautéing and browning. This can save up to 14 grams of fat for each tablespoon of fat not used. If you brown meat in a very hot cast-iron or nonstick pan, you may not need to use oil at all.

◆

Allow fat to drain off roasts by cooking on a rack.

◆

Separate the fat from the drippings before making gravy.

(See *Entertaining: Dinner Parties and Holiday Meals*, page 182, for a low-fat gravy recipe.)

◆

Drain pan-fried foods on paper towels before serving. Place cooked ground beef crumbles in a colander and rinse with hot water after draining to remove 2 to 5 grams of fat per 3-ounce serving.

◆

Always trim fat from meat and poultry before cooking to reduce the amount of fat that cooks into it.

◆

It's okay to leave the skin on poultry while cooking to keep the meat moist. Just be sure to remove it before eating to save up to 5 grams of fat per 3-ounce portion.

◆

Rather than pan-frying or deep-frying poultry or seafood, try oven-frying. Dip the skinless poultry or seafood in skim milk, then coat with seasoned bread crumbs or cornmeal and bake. Enjoy these oven-fried entrées instead of fish sticks or chicken strips to save about 5 grams of fat per 3-ounce serving.

◆

Marinades without oil tenderize lean cuts of meat as well as those with oil. It's the acidic ingredients, such as citrus juice, vinegar, or wine, that do the tenderizing. For a quick marinade, use a fat-free salad dressing. Or make your favorite marinade without the oil—you won't notice the difference.

All-Purpose Marinade

Combine ½ cup of orange juice; 1 teaspoon of honey; 1 teaspoon each of garlic powder, onion powder, and tarragon; and ½ teaspoon of black pepper. Pour over the meat or poultry and let sit from 20 minutes to overnight in the refrigerator.

◆

Combine lean ground beef and lean ground turkey breast or add a grain such as oatmeal or bread crumbs to reduce the fat in meatloaf, meatballs, burgers, or chili. Use egg whites or egg substitute in place of whole eggs to help hold the ground meat and grain together.

Fruit Salsa

Chop 1 melon (or 2 mangoes) and 1 large tomato (seeded) into small chunks. Add ⅓ cup of minced red onion; 1 clove of garlic, minced; and 2 tablespoons of fresh lime juice. Toss together and chill. Stir in 2 tablespoons of chopped, fresh cilantro or mint before serving. For extra sweetness, add 1 to 2 teaspoons of honey. For spiciness, add ½ jalapeno pepper, finely minced.

◆

Top fish or chicken with chutney or fruit salsa instead of a butter- or cream-based sauce before baking and save up to 19 grams of fat per quarter cup.

Mango Apricot Chutney

Chop a large mango and add 1 cup of diced dried apricots, 1 cup of onion, 1 tablespoon of fresh ginger, 2 cloves of garlic, ½ cup of brown sugar, 1 teaspoon of cloves, ½ teaspoon of red pepper flakes, and ½ cup of water. Simmer 1 hour.

◆

For moist, lower-fat chicken or fish dishes, wrap skinless chicken breasts or fish in parchment paper or foil along with vegetables, seasonings, and a small amount of wine or broth, then bake.

◆

Slice meat on an angle and fan it out on the plate to make a small portion look twice as large.

◆

Accompany your fish with a tablespoon of cocktail sauce, rather than tartar sauce, and save up to 8 grams of fat.

◆

Make fat-free sauces for meat, poultry, or seafood by puréeing cooked vegetables with a small amount of defatted broth or wine and seasonings.

Pastas, Sauces, and Stir-fries

If a recipe calls for tossing pasta in an oil mixture, substitute defatted broth.

◆

Serve pasta with marinara sauce and steamed vegetables for a low-fat meal.

◆

Make a hearty spaghetti sauce with meaty-textured vegetables, including eggplant, sun-dried tomatoes, and portobello mushrooms.

◆

To make a low-fat Alfredo sauce, use low-fat cottage or ricotta cheese blended with skim milk (rather than the cream found in most recipes) to a fine, smooth consistency.

◆

For other cream sauces, use buttermilk thickened with cornstarch (1 tablespoon of cornstarch for each cup of buttermilk) instead of cream or whole milk and save at least 6 grams of fat per cup.

cut the fat!

◆

When stir-frying, use lesser amounts of flavorful oils like sesame, chili, or herb-flavored, rather than the usual amounts of regular, less flavorful oils. You'll get more flavor with less fat.

◆

Use small amounts of lean meat or poultry in stir-fries. Slice the meat or poultry across the grain into thin strips and marinate before stir-frying. Thin slices allow the marinade to tenderize more of the meat.

Vegetables and Side Dishes

Sauté vegetables in a small amount of broth or fruit juice, in place of oil or butter. Season with herbs and spices.

◆

Sprinkle steamed vegetables with lemon pepper seasoning or imitation butter flakes or spray, rather than a teaspoon of margarine or butter, and save 4 grams of fat.

◆

Serve a baked potato instead of 10 french fries to save at least 8 grams of fat. Or make your own baked french fries for about one-third the fat of regular french fries.

Baked French Fries

Slice potatoes into uniformly sized wedges and toss with about 1 teaspoon of vegetable oil per potato and desired seasonings, such as rosemary with a dash of cayenne and salt. Bake at 475° for about 20 minutes, turning occasionally.

---

cut the fat!

◆

Use nonfat yogurt, nonfat sour cream, or an herbed nonfat or low-fat cottage cheese mixture instead of regular sour cream (2.5 grams of fat per tablespoon) or butter (12 grams of fat per tablespoon) on that baked potato.

Herbed Cottage Cheese

Blend together 1 cup of 1% cottage cheese (use nonfat cottage cheese for even less fat), 1 tablespoon of skim milk, 1 teaspoon of lemon juice, 1 tablespoon of chopped fresh parsley, and any combination of your favorite herbs and seasonings, such as basil and oregano, garlic and thyme, red pepper flakes and onion, roasted peppers and sun-dried tomatoes—the possibilities are endless! Use this as a tasty topping on baked potatoes or steamed vegetables or as a creamy dip for raw vegetables, crackers, and baked chips.

◆

Reduce or eliminate the margarine, butter, or oil called for in prepared rice and pasta mixes.

Other Mixed Dishes

Plan a meatless meal, such as low-fat cheese enchiladas, once or twice a week.

Cheese Enchiladas

Fill a soft corn tortilla with 1 to 2 table-spoons of low-fat shredded cheese, salsa, and your choice of vegetables, like chopped onion, tomatoes, and green pepper. Roll the tortilla, place on a heat-resistant dish, and heat in a microwave or conventional oven until the cheese melts. If desired, top with a small amount of low-fat or nonfat sour cream and additional salsa. Serve with rice or fat-free beans.

◆

Fajitas (sautéed lean beef or skinless chicken and vegetables wrapped in soft tortillas) can make a low-fat meal. Just use nonfat sour cream as a topping and go easy on the guacamole.

◆

Have a thin-crust pizza topped with vegetables such as green pepper, onions, broccoli, mushrooms, spinach, and eggplant. Go easy on the cheese. If you want a meat topping, try Canadian bacon rather than pepperoni or sausage to save over 6 grams of fat per ounce.

DESSERTS

You don't need to eliminate desserts. Enjoy lower-fat desserts or smaller portions of rich desserts—often just a taste is enough. (For more dessert ideas, see *Entertaining: Dinner Parties and Holiday Meals,* page 180)

◆

Experiment with reducing the fat in your dessert recipes by one-third to one-half.

For this dessert	Use this much fat
Cakes and soft-drop cookies	No more than 2 tablespoons of fat per cup of flour
Muffins, quick breads, biscuits	No more than 1 to 2 tablespoons of fat per cup of flour
Piecrust	½ cup of margarine or shortening for 2 cups of flour

◆

Substitute evaporated skim milk in recipes that call for heavy cream to save up to a whopping 90 grams of fat per cup.

◆

Using skim milk or buttermilk in place of whole milk in pudding and cream pie recipes saves 7 to 8.5 grams of fat per cup.

◆

By toasting nuts for enhanced flavor, you can reduce the amount used in recipes. You'll save at least 14 grams of fat for every ounce of nuts you omit. One ounce of nuts is about 10 to 12 macadamia nuts, 14 walnut halves, 18 medium cashews, 22 almonds, or 31 large pecans.

◆

Make a graham cracker piecrust using half oil and half fruit juice instead of melted butter or margarine.

◆

Top desserts with frozen low-fat vanilla yogurt instead of whipping cream.

◆

Make a chocolate sauce with evaporated skim milk, sugar, and powdered cocoa. To thicken, heat until almost boiling and add a small amount of cornstarch dissolved in cold water.

◆

Bake or poach fruit with cinnamon, cloves, honey, or sugar.

◆

For a frozen treat, choose fat-free or low-fat yogurt or ice cream (0 to 6 grams of fat per cup), sherbet or sorbet (usually less than 4 grams of fat), frozen fruit pops or popsicles (0 grams of fat), or Italian ices (0 grams of fat) in place of higher-fat ice cream (at least 15 grams of fat) desserts.

◆

For an occasional chocolate treat, make a low-fat chocolate fondue. Use fresh fruits such as strawberries, bananas, apples, oranges, and pineapple as dippers.

Chocolate Fondue

Stir together ¾ cup of sugar, ½ cup of unsweetened cocoa powder, and 4 teaspoons of cornstarch in a small saucepan. Add ⅔ cup of evaporated skim milk and cook over medium heat until thick and bubbly. Continue cooking for 2 minutes, stirring constantly. Take care not to cook too fast or at too high a temperature, or the sauce can become lumpy. And handle carefully, as the bubbling sauce is hotter than boiling water! Dip fresh strawberries, pineapple chunks, banana chunks, or grapes into the warm chocolate. Just 4 grams of fat in the entire recipe!

◆

Top angel food cake with a fat-free dessert glaze, fresh fruit, or fruit preserves for a fat-free, flavorful, and nutritious treat.

Fat-Free Dessert Glaze

Mix powdered sugar and enough water to make a glaze that slowly runs off the back of a spoon. *Hint:* Start with a very small amount of liquid and slowly add more to reach the desired consistency. For a more flavorful glaze, substitute lemon, orange, or lime juice as the liquid or add cocoa powder, cinnamon, dried orange or lemon rind, nutmeg, almond extract, or your favorite spice.

◆

Try a "skinny" fruit cobbler and save at least 3 grams of fat per serving compared with traditional fruit cobbler.

"Skinny" Fruit Cobbler

Put sliced fresh, frozen, or canned (drained) apples, peaches, blueberries, or raspberries in a nonstick baking pan coated lightly with vegetable oil cooking spray. (For best results, bake and serve in individual oven-safe bowls.) Sprinkle with low-fat cereal, brown sugar, and spices such as cinnamon, nutmeg, allspice, and ginger. Bake at 350° for 15 to 20 minutes. Top each serving with a dollop of low-fat or regular vanilla frozen yogurt.

◆

Rice pudding and tapioca can be made low-fat using egg whites or egg substitute and evaporated skim milk.

◆

Consider flavored gelatin with no fat as a dessert. For extra flair, add fresh fruit chunks and minimarshmallows.

◆

Finish your meal with gingersnaps, fruit bars, or vanilla wafers, which contain about 1 gram of fat apiece. Fortune cookies are usually fat-free.

BEVERAGES

If you haven't already, make the switch to skim or 1% milk. Over a 4-month period, gradually change from whole milk to 2%, then 1%, and finally skim. You can mix two types for a while to ease the transition. If you don't like the consistency of skim milk, try adding 1 to 2 tablespoons of nonfat dry milk powder to 1 cup of skim milk to give it more "body" without adding any fat.

◆

Flavored coffees are tasty alternatives to richer coffee mixes. If you usually add half-and-half or light cream to your coffee, try evaporated or powdered skim milk to save 2 to 3 grams of fat per tablespoon.

◆

Hooked on cappuccino, latte, or café mocha? Order these with skim milk instead of whole milk to save about 8 grams of fat.

◆

Enjoy a cup of hot apple cider instead of hot cocoa and save over 3 grams of fat. Or have a low-fat hot cocoa made with skim milk or a low-fat mix.

◆

To save about 9 grams of fat per cup, make a milk shake with skim milk or nonfat yogurt instead of whole milk and ice cream. Add ice cubes and fruit (strawberries, raspberries, banana) or chocolate syrup.

◆

Cream-based liqueurs contain up to 5 grams of fat per ounce. If you're choosing an after-dinner liqueur, opt for those that are not cream based.

Depending on your total daily calorie intake, the extra calories from alcoholic beverages may be stored in your body as fat. To trim potential fat calories, limit the number of alcoholic beverages you drink and try lower-calorie alcoholic beverages, like wine spritzers and light beer. If you choose to drink alcoholic beverages, limit yourself to 1 or 2 drinks a day.

SNACKS

Reduced-fat potato chips contain 7 grams of fat per ounce—3 grams less than regular chips. There are also fat-free chips available. Pretzels usually contain 1 gram of fat or less per ounce.

◆

Enjoy baked tortilla chips (13 chips contain only 1 gram of fat) with salsa or fat-free bean dip, which—compared with higher-fat dips like guacamole—can save you up to 5 grams of fat per 1-ounce serving. You can also make your own chips from bagels, pita bread, and potatoes.

Baked Chips

Bagels: Thinly slice a whole, uncut bagel into little rounds.

Pita bread: Separate the pita into halves and cut into quarters.

Tortillas: Slice soft corn or flour tortillas into quarters.

Potatoes: Slice small potatoes with the skin on into thin slices.

Place flat on a pan and spray lightly with vegetable oil cooking spray. If desired, sprinkle with garlic powder, butter-flavored granules, or your favorite herb. Bake in a 400° oven until crisp, about 10 minutes.

◆

Rice cakes of any flavor or variety have no fat. Melba toast and soda crackers are also good low-fat crunchy snacks.

◆

Top toasted raisin bread with apple butter or a thin layer of reduced-fat peanut butter (1 tablespoon has about 6 grams of fat).

◆

Try air-popped popcorn. For added flavor, sprinkle with grated Parmesan or Romano cheese (about 1.5 grams of fat per table-spoon) and your favorite seasonings. If you're in a hurry, choose microwave pop-corn with less than 3 grams of fat per cup in the plain or light varieties.

◆

Cut up raw vegetables, such as carrots, zucchini, and peppers, or use precut packaged vegetables for a fast, low-fat, nutritious snack. Dip in salsa, plain nonfat yogurt with dried dill or basil, or low-fat or nonfat ranch salad dressing.

◆

Make your own fat-free flavored spread and serve with breads, crackers, and raw fruits and vegetables.

Fat-Free Spreads

Start with 8 ounces of softened nonfat cream cheese. Add the following ingredients and mix until incorporated:

Orange-spiked: Add the zest of 1 orange and 2 tablespoons of orange juice.

Lemon-infused: Add the zest of 1 lemon and 2 teaspoons of lemon juice.

Garlic-herb: Add 1 clove of minced garlic, 1 teaspoon of dried basil or thyme leaves, and pepper.

Italian-herb: Add 1 packet of Italian salad dressing mix.

Honey-mustard: Add 1 packet of honey-mustard salad dressing mix.

Mock-caramel: Add ¾ cup of brown sugar, ¼ cup of white sugar, and 2 teaspoons of vanilla.

◆

A bowl of whole-grain cereal with skim or low-fat milk makes a great low-fat (less than 5 grams), high-fiber snack.

◆

To make a low-fat pizza snack, spread 1 to 2 tablespoons of pizza or tomato sauce on a plain English muffin. Add 1 ounce of shredded low-fat mozzarella cheese and sliced or cut-up vegetables, such as onions, green peppers, and mushrooms. Heat until the cheese melts.

◆

Want something fast and hot? Heat low-fat soup or chili in the microwave.

cut the fat!

◆

For sweet snack attacks, choose "light" varieties of snack cakes and cupcakes and save at least half the fat of regular varieties, as well as one-third the calories.

◆

When a cookie craving strikes, instead of two ½-ounce chunky chocolate chip cookies at 10 grams of fat, consider two graham crackers or two fig bars, each containing 2 grams of fat. Other low-fat cookies include gingersnaps, fruit bars, vanilla wafers, and animal crackers. Look for reduced-fat versions of your favorites.

◆

Fat-free (but not calorie-free!) candy choices include black or red licorice, marshmallows, most hard candies, gummy candies, and jelly beans.

◆

Don't forget fresh fruit as a fast snack. Try different fruits for a change, such as pineapple, papaya, and mango. Frozen fruit chunks, such as grapes or banana slices, also make a tasty and refreshing snack.

◆

Raisins and other dried fruits, such as apples, apricots, pineapple, and bananas, are healthful, low-fat snack foods. Fruit rolls can also make low-fat snacks; most varieties have no more than 1 gram of fat per roll.

◆

Grab a snack cup of low-fat pudding or yogurt. For added crunch, sprinkle on dry cereal.

◆

For low-fat frozen snacks, make your own popsicles from fruit juice or enjoy store-bought fat-free frozen treats, including fruit juice bars and Italian ice. Other low-fat options include frozen yogurt bars and frozen yogurt.

◆

Reach for a frozen banana instead of a cup of ice cream and save at least 14 grams of fat.

◆

Make your own low-fat ice cream sandwich using low-fat frozen yogurt or ice cream and graham crackers or vanilla wafers. Or scoop into a plain ice cream cone, which contains virtually no fat.

◆

For a fat-free, icy snack beverage, blend skim milk or fruit juice with frozen strawberries or banana chunks and ½ teaspoon of honey or sugar.

Quick "Pick-Me-Up" Shake

Blend together 1 frozen banana or 2 cups of frozen strawberries (or half of each) with 1 to 1½ cups of apple or orange juice or skim milk. If using skim milk, chocolate lovers could add 1 tablespoon of sugar and 2 teaspoons of cocoa. *Hint:* To freeze a banana, peel when just ripe, chop if desired, place in airtight plastic freezer bag, and freeze.

◆

For another quick and cold refresher, purée peaches, strawberries, or blueberries with cinnamon and some sugar and spoon over low-fat frozen yogurt or low-fat vanilla yogurt.

◆

Update the root beer float using ½ cup of low-fat ice cream and 1 cup (8 ounces) of root beer for a beverage with no more than 3 grams of fat.

Eating Out

Full-Service Restaurants

Use your knowledge of low-fat foods and preparation methods to help limit your fat intake when eating out. Enjoy the luxury of someone else preparing your meal and serving you—even allow yourself to splurge occasionally—but try to set limits on higher-fat choices if you eat out frequently.

BREAKFAST

Substitute 2 ounces of 2% milk for half-and-half in your coffee and save about 6 grams of fat. Replace the 2% milk with skim and save another gram of fat for each cup of coffee.

◆

Try chewing instead of drinking your morning fruit. Whole, fresh, or canned fruit provides not only more fiber and chewing satisfaction, but also a "full feeling" to help you eat fewer higher-fat foods.

◆

There is a "sunny side" to eggs. Egg whites and most egg substitutes have no fat. Order these scrambled or as an omelet in place of a 3-egg omelet and save about 15 grams of fat.

◆

Request that eggs be cooked with vegetable oil cooking spray instead of butter or margarine.

◆

Order your toast or English muffin without butter or margarine. Use a fruit spread, like orange marmalade, strawberry jelly, or preserves, and save 4 grams of fat for every teaspoon of butter or margarine you don't use.

◆

Three medium slices of bacon or 3 links of sausage will add 9 to 12 grams of fat to your breakfast. Try lower-fat versions or request lean ham or Canadian bacon as a lower-fat substitute.

APPETIZERS

Begin your meal with a broth-based soup as an appetizer and you will be less likely to overindulge for the rest of your meal.

◆

Also start your meal with a glass of water to help to curb your appetite.

◆

Go easy on the bread basket, especially if your eyes are bigger than your stomach. While bread is very low in fat and sometimes fat-free, it does contain calories. Adding butter or margarine adds 4 grams of fat per teaspoon. If you're likely to fill up on bread and butter before your meal, ask that the bread be served with the meal or not at all.

◆

The term "loaded" in menu descriptions often means a load of fat. "Loaded" potato skins and nachos are two higher-fat appetizer choices. Split these with several people or, better yet, go for the bread and cracker basket as a lower-fat option.

◆

Think twice before gobbling up the "wild" or BBQ chicken wings and fingers. Remove the high-fat skin on chicken wings and there's not much left to gobble. Chicken fingers start out as lean meat and become a high-fat appetizer after being fried. If you're in the mood for poultry, skip the high-fat appetizers and choose grilled chicken as your entrée.

◆

Go easy on the basket of tortilla chips. Each chip can contain up to 1 gram of fat! If a basket of tortilla chips is served when you sit down, put a small amount of chips on your plate and then ask that the basket be removed. If you do finish the basket, ask that it not be refilled. Load up on salsa, though—it's fat-free.

LUNCH AND DINNER

Look for what can be substituted or swapped on the menu. Perhaps one entrée is served on a bed of spinach. If you want the spinach but a different entrée, try ordering the spinach with the entrée you want.

◆

Ask for heavy sauces, butter, sour cream, and salad dressings "on the side." This way you have control over how much you eat. Be aware, though, that large amounts are sometimes served this way, so control your urge to add more than you need.

◆

Try enjoying the natural flavors of food without butter- or cream-based sauces. Just ¼ cup of hollandaise, béarnaise, or Alfredo sauce can add 17 to 19 grams of fat. Tomato-based sauces are fine; steak and soy sauces have no fat.

◆

Plan ahead for a special lunch or dinner. If you know you'll want to splurge, eat smaller, lower-fat meals beforehand. Consider drinking a glass of fruit or tomato juice about a half hour before going to the restaurant to help curb your appetite.

◆

Have an idea of what you would like to eat before looking at the menu—or even before you enter the restaurant.

Look for these words in menu descriptions as clues to lower-fat selections:

Grilled	Charbroiled
Poached	Boiled
Baked	Barbecued
Broiled	Mesquite-grilled
Roasted	Garden-fresh
Steamed	Broth
Stir-fried	Au jus
Rotisserie	Marinated in juice or
Flame-broiled	wine

◆

If you're not sure how a food item is prepared, just ask. Then you can order by choice, not by chance.

◆

Special orders shouldn't upset anyone. If you would like your meal prepared differently, don't hesitate to ask. And send it back if you didn't get what you ordered.

These words in menu descriptions are clues to higher-fat selections:

Creamed or creamy	Flaky
	In its own gravy
Puffed	Hollandaise
Crispy	Alfredo
Battered	À la king
Breaded	Béarnaise
Pan-fried	Mornay
Au gratin	Scampi
Cheese sauce	Marinated in oil or
Buttery	butter

◆

Ask for a "doggie bag" at the beginning of your meal and stow away the food you don't plan to eat to enjoy another day.

◆

Split it! If you know the entrée is much larger than you need (which is typical in many restaurants), split your main meal with your dining companion. Round out the meal with extra vegetables or a house salad with dressing "on the side."

◆

Ask for the lunch portion or half portion, even if it is dinner. "Half portion" means half the fat.

◆

Create a custom meal at just about any restaurant by ordering side dishes. A satisfying and delicious meal with plenty of variety and color can easily be created this way. For instance, order 1 vegetable side, 1 rice side, a dinner roll, a vegetable-based soup, and fruit with frozen yogurt or 1 scoop of regular ice cream for dessert.

◆

Just because your favorite menu item says "fried" or "sautéed in butter" doesn't mean the chef can prepare it only that way. Ask for the meal to be prepared without added fats and let the chef be creative!

DESSERTS

If you have your eye on pie, keep these numbers in mind: ⅛ of a pecan pie contains about 24 grams of fat; ⅛ of a chocolate cream pie about 17 grams of fat; and ⅛ of an apple pie about 14 grams of fat.

◆

Because fat lurks in the piecrust, go easy on double-crusted pies. Choose ⅛ of a single-crust pie and save 7 grams of fat.

◆

Order an ice cream alternative. Sherbets, sorbets, Italian ices, and frozen yogurts are almost always lower in fat than ice cream. And they can be just as satisfying!

◆

Go bananas . . . or any other fruit for dessert. Just about any seasonal fruit can be ordered for dessert at many restaurants. Fruit is virtually fat-free!

◆

Consider splitting that slice of cheesecake—the more people the better. One-eighth of a 9-inch cheesecake can contain more than 20 grams fat.

◆

If you really want it, have it. There is no such word as "NEVER" when it comes to dessert! Plan ahead by choosing lower-fat foods and increasing your physical activity. If the dessert was not planned, try to make up for it by eating lower-fat meals and increasing your activity over the next day or two.

Quick-Service Restaurants, Delis, and Cafés

Ask for nutrition information (posted or printed in pamphlets at most quick-service restaurants) to help you make an informed choice about low-fat fast-food options. And consider going "light." Many fast-food restaurants are now offering reduced-fat menu items.

BREAKFAST

Consider this before ordering a breakfast sandwich: a sausage, egg, and cheese croissant sandwich has 40 grams of fat. Replace the croissant with an English muffin and save 13 grams of fat, or choose Canadian bacon, egg, and cheese on an English muffin and save 29 grams of fat.

◆

Choose your muffins carefully. Jumbo muffins can contain more fat than many doughnuts. Opt for half a muffin or a low-fat or fat-free muffin instead.

◆

Bagel shop bagels usually contain 1 to 2 grams of fat. Smear on 2 tablespoons of cream cheese and you add 10 grams of fat. Try light cream cheese at half the fat of regular cream cheese or, if available, fat-free cream cheese or jelly at 0 grams of fat.

◆

Rather than a custard-filled éclair at 12 grams of fat, choose a lower-fat doughnut, such as a glazed doughnut at 7 grams of fat. Better yet, choose a bagel to save about 10 grams of fat.

◆

Pancake or waffle breakfasts are low-fat options. Top with syrup and skip the butter to keep them low-fat.

◆

Don't forget that cereal and skim or low-fat milk is a low-fat choice when grabbing a quick breakfast.

LUNCH AND DINNER

At the salad, taco, or potato bar, use a smaller plate so you can't stack as much food on it. This can help limit the calories and fat you consume.

◆

Choose low-fat or nonfat dressing at the salad bar, or make your own dressing with fresh lemon and vinegar.

◆

While salad bars are filled with greens, watch out for the fat traps, like salad dressings (up to 9 grams of fat per tablespoon), croutons (5 grams of fat per ounce), shredded cheddar cheese (5 grams of fat per 2 tablespoons), bacon bits (about 2 grams of fat per tablespoon), and creamy salads like potato salad (up to 9 grams of fat per ¼ cup). A low-fat salad includes plenty of greens and is topped with alfalfa sprouts, broccoli, carrots, cucumbers, artichoke hearts, mushrooms, onions, and peppers. A 75–100-grams-of-fat (way over par!) salad can become a satisfying and delicious 5–10-grams-of-fat salad with some smart choices.

◆

Low-fat toppings for your burger include lettuce, onion, pickles, salsa, mustard, and ketchup. Choose these toppings rather than cheese and save about 4 grams of fat per slice of cheese.

◆

Corned beef on rye bread with mustard is a low-fat alternative to a Reuben.

◆

Select broiled, rotisserie, baked, or barbecued chicken instead of fried or breaded. Remove the skin before you eat it and save up to 5 grams of fat for a 3-ounce piece of chicken (the size of a small breast).

◆

Go easy on the avocado or guacamole on salads and Mexican dishes. Half an avocado has about 15 grams of fat.

◆

Ask for your food without special sauces, toppings, and dressings to help reduce the fat. Hold the mayonnaise to save 11 grams of fat for every tablespoon. But keep the mustard. It takes 2 tablespoons of mustard to add up to just 1 gram of fat. And ketchup is fat-free!

◆

Don't be fooled by the cost savings of jumbo meals. Think of your fat savings instead. Choose regular fries at about 12 grams of fat a serving in place of the large fries to save over 6 grams of fat. Imagine how much fat you could save over a year!

In just one year, it's possible to save up to a whopping 1000 fat grams by eating just one fewer serving of large fries a week!

◆

Some low-fat-sounding foods, such as taco salad, chicken sandwich, or chicken club, can actually be loaded with fat. A taco salad served in a fried shell can contain over 60 grams of fat, a breaded, fried chicken sandwich can contain as much as 40 grams, and a chicken club ("club" = added bacon and mayonnaise) can contain as much as 24 grams.

◆

Say "No cheese!" If bone-building calcium is what you want, round out your meal by ordering nonfat or low-fat milk or frozen yogurt rather than cheese. Save cheese for places (like home) where you can opt for lower-fat varieties.

◆

Low in fat is not synonymous with "all you can eat." If your favorite fast-food item has only 5 grams of fat, it will become 25 grams if you eat five servings.

◆

Choose grilled or sliced meat sandwiches, rather than fried or breaded.

◆

Submarine sandwiches can be low in fat if you choose lean meats and lots of vegetables without extra creamy sauces and spreads. And stick to the 6-inch size.

◆

Go for the regular hamburger with no more than 12 grams of fat, instead of the quarter-pound (large) burger with 23 grams, double burger with 27 grams, or triple burger with 42 grams.

◆

Accompany your meal with a plain baked potato or a side salad with fat-free dressing, rather than fries or onion rings, and save up to 24 grams of fat.

◆

Choose a grilled chicken sandwich without mayonnaise (about 10 fat grams) instead of a fried chicken sandwich and save at least 14 fat grams. Similar savings apply to fish sandwiches.

◆

If chicken is your choice, an extra-crisp fried thigh at 30 grams of fat is one of the highest-fat chicken selections around. For leaner alternatives, try a rotisserie roasted chicken breast with the wing and save up to 12 grams of fat, or a rotisserie roasted chicken breast without the skin or wing (the leanest choice) and save up to 26 grams of fat.

◆

Order white meat poultry rather than dark. Dark meat can have three times as much fat as white meat.

◆

Select thin-crust pizza, order with half the cheese, and load up on the vegetables, like green peppers, hot peppers, broccoli, spinach, onions, tomatoes, and mushrooms.

DESSERTS

Mmm, mmm, milk shakes! These dairy desserts can be as high as 14 grams of fat for a small serving or as low as 1 gram of fat for a low-fat milk shake. Check the nutrition information or ask your food server if the milk shakes are low in fat.

♦

Even though filled with fruit, dessert snack pies contain about 15 grams of fat. To satisfy a sweet tooth, have a vanilla frozen yogurt cone at less than 1 gram of fat or a frozen yogurt sundae with 1 to 3 grams of fat and save over 12 grams of fat.

Eating Out Ethnic

Enjoy the variety of food choices available when eating out ethnic. Use this guide to find delicious, low-fat options on ethnic menus. Look for key words as clues to lower-fat finds, and don't hesitate to ask your servers about preparation techniques or for special requests.

CAJUN

Lower-Fat Finds	Fat Traps
Appetizer/Side:	*Appetizer/Side:*
Red beans and rice, Cajun rice, Candied yams, Greens, Cornbread (without butter)	Dirty rice, Bisques and étouffées
Main dish:	*Main dish:*
Jambalaya or gumbo (with poultry or seafood), Blackened or baked fish, Boiled seafood dishes	Dishes with andouille or boudin, Deep-fried seafood or poultry

CARIBBEAN

Lower-Fat Finds

Appetizer/Side:

Black bean or chicken soup, Okra, Baked pawpaw

Main dish:

Jerk meats; Broiled, grilled, steamed, or boiled seafood; Red beans and rice; Rice with pork; Shrimp and rice; Stuffed fish; Fruit sauces served with dish

Fat Traps

Appetizer/Side:

Coconut, Cream-based soups or bisque

Main dish:

Conch fritters; Meat, seafood, or poultry poached in coconut milk; Baked snapper with green sauce; Beef with eggplant; Cabbage with corned beef; Duckling with pineapple; Stuffed cheese with meat or seafood filling *cut the fat!*

CHINESE

Lower-Fat Finds	**Fat Traps**
Appetizer/Side:	*Appetizer/Side:*
Vegetable, hot-and-sour, or chicken wonton soup; Drunken chicken; Steamed dumplings; Steamed rice	Spring or egg rolls, Fried wontons, Fried dumplings (Pot stickers), Sesame noodles, Fried rice
Main dish:	*Main dish:*
Black bean sauce on fish, Stir-fried foods (if light on the oil or steamed instead) such as Moo Goo Gai Pan	Peking duck, Fried meat or poultry dishes (like General Tsao's chicken, Lemon chicken, and Sweet-and-sour pork or chicken), Dishes with nuts such as Cashew chicken

EASTERN EUROPEAN

Lower-Fat Finds	**Fat Traps**
Appetizer/Side:	*Appetizer/Side:*
Stuffed cabbage or peppers (with rice), Yogurt-based borscht or fruit soups, Knishes filled with vegetables	Blintz, Tomatoes nana
Main dish:	*Main dish:*
Poached fish or poultry	Beef goulash, Chicken fricassee, Chicken paprika, Schnitzel, Sausages (including kielbasa)

FRENCH

Lower-Fat Finds	**Fat Traps**
Appetizer/Side:	*Appetizer/Side:*
Seafood bouillabaisse, Salad Niçoise (if light on dressing), Baguette, Purée of rice and turnips, Spinach braised with onions	Croissants, Cassoulets, Gratins, Fish stew with mayonnaise, Cream soups (such as cream of onion)
Main dish:	*Main dish:*
Roast chicken (without the skin), Seafood dishes (if poached, steamed, oven-roasted, or seared), Sauces served with entrées like coulis (if no cream used) or vegetable purée	Quenelles, Soufflés, Poached chicken with cheese sauce, Chicken in a cold dish, Stuffed beef roll, Sauces served with entrée like hollandaise, béarnaise, or beurre blanc

GREEK

Lower-Fat Finds	Fat Traps
Appetizer/Side:	*Appetizer/Side:*
Grilled vegetable skewers; Chicken rice, lentil, or chickpea soup; Pita bread	Taramasalata, Stuffed pastries like bourekakia, Tomato salad with feta cheese, Fried cheese (saganaki), Spanikopita (spinach pie)
Main dish:	*Main dish:*
Shish kebabs or souvlaki made with lamb, beef, poultry, seafood, or vegetables; Roast lamb	Pastitsio, Meats with egg-based lemon sauce called avgolemono

INDIAN

Lower-Fat Finds

Appetizer/Side:

Chipati, Biryani (vegetable or seafood), Curried chickpeas, Fruit salad with thickened milk, Lentils and spinach, Naan, Rice with chickpeas or peas, Vegetable curry, Lentil or split pea soups, Chutney

Main dish:

Bhuna (fish or lamb); Chicken or fish prepared in tikka-, vindaloo-, or masala-style; Curried chicken (if yogurt based)

Fat Traps

Appetizer/Side:

Fried appetizers or breads like samosas, pakoras, poori, paratha; Rice cooked in coconut milk

Main dish:

Dishes with labels such as kandhari, malai, and korma; Beef or chicken cooked in coconut milk

ITALIAN

Lower-Fat Finds	**Fat Traps**
Appetizer/Side:	*Appetizer/Side:*
Pasta e fagioli, Minestrone soup, Marinated calamari, Steamed clams	Meat and cheese antipasto, Fritto misto, Garlic bread, Shrimp and vegetable salad (made with oil and mayonnaise)
Main dish:	*Main dish:*
Chicken or veal cacciatore; Cioppino; Pasta with tomato- (marinara) or wine-based sauce; Marinara dishes; Primavera dishes; Stewed squid with tomatoes and peas; Linguini (or spaghetti) with eggplant or red clam sauce; Grilled veal, fish, game, or chicken	Cheese-filled canelloni, tortellini, lasagna, and ravioli; Pesto and cream-based sauces, like Alfredo and carbonara; Risotto; Veal or chicken parmigiana; Italian sausage; Spaghetti with garlic and oil

JAPANESE

Lower-Fat Finds

Appetizer/Side:

Miso soup, Chicken in rice cake soup, Clams and scallions in bean soup, Chicken and noodles in miso soup, White turnips in bean soup, Beef and potato stew, Peas and rice, Red rice and beans, Sweet simmered oriental vegetables

Main dish:

Teriyaki or sukiyaki; Sushi; Pinecone squid; Sashimi; Fish and noodle casserole; Cold steamed chicken; Fish steaks; Grilled scallops, chicken, or shrimp

Fat Traps

Appetizer/Side:

Tempura (Agemono), Glazed grilled chicken wings

Main dish:

Egg dishes like Oyako-donburi

MEXICAN/ SOUTHWESTERN

Lower-Fat Finds

Appetizer/Side:

Black beans or black bean soup, Cantaloupe soup, Ceviche, Corn or flour tortillas, Gazpacho, Salsa, Pot beans, Tortilla soup

Main dish:

Arroz con pollo; Vegetable, bean, chicken, or beef burrito; Fajitas; Soft taco; Mesquite-grilled chicken, seafood, or lean meat

Fat Traps

Appetizer/Side:

Nachos, Tortilla chips, Guacamole, Taco salads in shell, Refried beans, Avocado soup

Main dish:

Chimichangas, Flautas, Taquitos, Tamales, Quesadillas, Cheese enchiladas, Chile con queso, Chile rellenos, Huevos rancheros, Cilantro pesto or poblano aioli served with meal

MIDDLE EASTERN

Lower-Fat Finds	**Fat Traps**
Appetizer/Side:	*Appetizer/Side:*
Couscous, Baba ghanoush, Hummus (when light on the olive oil and tahini), Dolma (Stuffed grape leaves), Lentil soup, Pita bread, Rice pilaf, Tabouleh, Fattoush	Hummus (when heavy on olive oil and tahini)
Main dish:	*Main dish:*
Kofta	Falafel, Kasseri, Kibbee, Meat pies

SPANISH

Lower-Fat Finds	Fat Traps
Appetizer/Side:	*Appetizer/Side:*
Tapas—Spanish appetizers, such as escageche, gazpacho, or chicharron de gallina	Aceitunas, Jamon serrano
Main dish:	*Main dish:*
Paella made with seafood, pork, or chicken; Fish or chicken baked in picada sauce	Tortilla española, Chorizo salteado

THAI

Lower-Fat Finds	**Fat Traps**

Appetizer/Side:

Pad thai, Corn and shrimp soup, Crystal noodle, Papaya and shrimp salad, Seafood kabob, Shrimp and orange chili salad, Squid salad, Steamed mussels, Sweet-and-sour cucumber, Steamed rice, Plain fried rice

Appetizer/Side:

Coconut-based soups and curries, Peanut sauce, Pork and chicken stew

Main dish:

Garlic shrimp, Thai chicken, Seafood platter, Scallops bamboo, Sautéed ginger beef or chicken (if light on oil when sautéed)

Main dish:

Deep-fried dishes like Royal tofu and Hot thai catfish, Red beef or Green chicken curry

On the Go

In this fast-paced world, we often find ourselves grabbing a quick meal or snack on the go. Use the tips in Eating Out *along with the ideas below for eating low-fat in various situations. Be prepared to bring lower-fat snacks and meals along with you whenever possible by shopping for easy-to-prepare and -transport low-fat foods.*

ON THE ROAD

A fast and economical alternative to eating out on the road is packing food to eat in the car or at rest stops along the way. Depending on how long you'll be driving and how many companions you'll have, you can pack a thermos, lunch bag, or cooler with lots of low-fat, nutritious foods.

◆

For a warm pick-me-up, bring along some coffee, tea, hot cocoa (made with 1% or skim milk), or soup in a thermos.

◆

Low-fat foods that don't need to be kept warm or cold include raw vegetables and fresh or dried fruits; low-fat or fat-free baked goods like cookies, muffins, bagels, and fruit bars; air-popped popcorn; and vacuum-packed low-fat puddings. Vacuum-packed fruit juices and canned and bottled beverages also don't need to be chilled.

◆

Snacks to keep chilled in a cooler include low-fat meat, sandwich spreads, and dairy products like skim or 1% milk and low-fat cheese and yogurt.

◆

Freeze juice boxes or cartons. They'll thaw in an hour or two for a cool thirst quencher.

IN THE AIR

If you're traveling by air, be sure to inquire at least 48 hours in advance about alternative menus. Airlines offer a variety of low-fat menus, but you'll have to ask a few questions to see what's included. Low-fat options may be called "heart-healthy," "fruit and salad," "vegetarian" (which may or may not be low-fat), "low-calorie," "low-cholesterol," "diabetic," and, of course, "low-fat."

◆

If you're flying on short notice and don't have time to order in advance, remember you don't *have* to clean your plate. Go lightly on the salad dressing, butter, or dessert.

◆

If the only snack offered is a high-fat item like peanuts, ask if pretzels might be available. Or consider bringing your own snack along.

◆

If you plan to eat soon after your plane lands, you could skip the airline food altogether.

ON THE JOB

Bring your own low-fat snacks to meetings.

◆

At a morning meeting, reach for a bagel with 1 tablespoon of cream cheese instead of a croissant and save 5 to 6 grams of fat.

◆

At the vending machine, choose pretzels instead of potato chips to save 9 grams of fat. Other low-fat vending machine alternatives include low-fat yogurt, fruit juice, pretzels, gummy fruit or licorice, and fresh fruit.

◆

Drink plenty of water or other nonfat or low-fat beverages such as water flavored with slices of fresh lemon, lime, or orange, fruit juice, or skim or 1% milk.

◆

Keep your desk drawer stocked with such items as instant vegetable soups and oatmeals, dried fruit, snack-size whole-grain cereal, minicans of water-packed tuna, and low-fat crackers.

◆

If you're planning a meeting where food will be served, be sure to have several lower-fat options available. For breakfast, include bagels, low-fat muffins, fruit, fruit spreads, and mixed dried fruit. For lunch, consider lean ham, lean roast beef, turkey, and tossed salad greens with low-fat dressing.

AT THE GAME OR SHOW

Select a soft pretzel with mustard for a warm, chewy snack that is lower in fat than peanuts or pizza.

◆

Peanuts in the shell are a fun snack, but remember that a couple handfuls can add up to about 14 grams of fat.

◆

Choose air-popped popcorn, if available, instead of oil-popped. For 3 cups, you'll save 8 grams of fat. And skip the added butter-flavor topping to save even more.

◆

Share your popcorn with a friend and save half the fat.

◆

If you prefer candies, select 10 large jelly beans or 1 ounce of hard candies (with 0 fat grams) or even 10 to 12 chocolate-coated raisins or mint snacks (1.5 to 3 grams of fat) over 10 chocolate-coated peanuts or a chocolate-coated nougat/caramel/nut bar (both contain about 13.5 grams of fat). If you decide on a bar, try chocolate with just nougat and caramel to save 4.5 grams, or chocolate with nougat only to save 5.5 fat grams.

◆

Select a fruit juice bar rather than an ice cream bar and save up to 25 grams of fat.

◆

Drink a diet soda, seltzer, or fruit juice instead of getting a snack.

Entertaining

Eating low-fat in social situations can be challenging. When hosting a party, do your guests a favor and be sure to offer plenty of lower-fat options. As a guest, practice the tips learned in other sections and enjoy the event!

IF YOU ARE THE HOST

CASUAL BUFFETS AND COOKOUTS

Instead of offering bowls of nuts as snacks, serve whole nuts in the shell—these take more work to eat, so guests will likely eat fewer. Better yet, make a trail mix with pretzels, dried fruits, cereals, and just a few chopped nuts.

◆

Offer low-fat or nonfat dips, such as salsa, nonfat bean dips, and nonfat yogurt or sour cream dips, with baked tortilla chips and fresh fruits and vegetables.

◆

Include healthful, high-flavor extras to liven up the meal. Use salsas, relishes, purées, and flavored oils and vinegars to top lean slices of sirloin, boneless, skinless chicken breast, white-flesh fish, or steamed shrimp.

◆

Start a buffet line with pasta and vegetable salads with low-fat dressings and fruit salads with nonfat yogurt for a topping.

◆

Offer lean cold cuts and low-fat cheeses with low-fat or nonfat condiments like mustard and relishes. Serve with sliced tomatoes, lettuce, sprouts, and green pepper rings. Whole-grain breads and rolls add a nutty taste.

◆

Serve a variety of pasta salads flavored with zesty and low- or reduced-fat herb dressings. Include lots of fresh, frozen, or canned vegetables in the salad for added nutrients, fiber, color, and flavor.

◆

A salad of greens, such as spinach, curly endive, radicchio, and red cabbage with a burst of summer fruit like grapes or berries, makes a delicious and colorful main course or side dish.

◆

Offer cut-up vegetables such as carrots; jicama; celery; broccoli; mushrooms; and red, green, and yellow peppers with hummus (see recipe for *Hummus* in *At Home—Lunch and Dinner,* page 74) or low-fat or nonfat ranch dressing.

◆

Include plenty of fresh fruit. Cut cantaloupe and watermelon wedges with the rind on for easy munching. Serve bowls of fresh grapes, blueberries, and strawberries to eat by the handful.

◆

Wrap corn on the cob in foil and grill for 10 minutes each side. Use a butter-flavored spray in place of margarine or butter and you could save about 10 grams of fat.

◆

Grill burgers made from lean ground beef, ground turkey breast, or a combination of the two.

◆

Skewer sweet and white potato quarters with quartered onion, sprinkle with paprika, and grill.

DINNER PARTIES AND HOLIDAY MEALS

Serve low-fat yogurt, low-fat cream cheese, skim-milk ricotta cheese, or salsa-based dips with fresh vegetables and baked chips (see recipe for *Baked Chips* in *At Home—Snacks*, page 107), bread sticks, or reduced-fat crackers.

◆

Offer a variety of cheeses, including reduced-fat selections.

◆

Steamed, fresh artichokes are wonderful appetizers for a small dinner party. Instead of melted butter or margarine, dip leaves into a nonfat sauce consisting of nonfat yogurt with either Dijon mustard and a dash of cayenne pepper or lemon juice and a dash of hot pepper sauce.

◆

Self-basting turkeys are injected with a buttery liquid. So serve an unbasted turkey (or ham, duck, or goose) and baste frequently with wine, fruit juice, or broth instead of drippings.

♦

Make low-fat gravy or use a low-fat gravy mix.

Low-Fat Gravy

Pour drippings from roasting pan into a glass measuring cup or gravy separator. The fat will float to the top and the flavorful juices will settle to the bottom. If using a measuring cup, remove the top layer of fat with a baster. If using a separator, pour the bottom layer of juices into a saucepan. Heat the juices until simmering. Add additional canned broth if a large quantity of gravy is needed. Meanwhile, add cornstarch or flour (1–2 tablespoons of cornstarch or ¼ cup of flour will thicken about 2 cups of liquid) to a small amount of cold water, wine, or broth. Mix until smooth. Slowly add this to the simmering juices, stirring constantly with a wire whisk. Bring to a boil for about 30 seconds. Continue heating until gravy thickens, about 3 to 5 minutes, and serve immediately.

HOLIDAY MENU MAKEOVER

Before	After
3 ounces roast duck	3 ounces roast turkey breast
½ cup stuffing	½ cup rice pilaf
½ cup broccoli with hollandaise sauce	½ cup broccoli with lemon juice
½ cup jellied cranberry sauce	½ cup fresh cranberry relish
1 medium crescent roll	1 medium dinner roll
1 slice pecan pie	1 slice pumpkin pie
Total calories = 1205	Total calories = 730
Total fat = 55 grams	Total fat = 21 grams

♦

Reduce the amount of margarine in stuffing recipes and replace with fruit juice, wine, vegetable or meat stock, or low-sodium broth that has been reduced by about one half. To reduce stock (or any liquid), simmer uncovered until approximately one-half to one-third the starting quantity is left. For extra flavor in stuffings, add roasted vegetables (like red peppers) and onions, leeks, celery, mushrooms, and fresh herbs that have been sautéed in broth or wine.

♦

Serve fresh breads or rolls such as sourdough or French bread with the meal instead of higher-fat breads like croissants or biscuits.

◆

Offer nonfat spreads for breads, such as apple butter or cranberry relish.

◆

When adding nuts to vegetable dishes or salads, toast them first to enhance the flavor and then use half the amount called for in the recipe.

◆

In place of buttered bread crumbs on casseroles, use crushed cereal flakes.

◆

Try adding balsamic vinegar or lemon juice and your favorite seasonings to cooked vegetables instead of butter or cream sauces.

◆

Offer several grain dishes with the meal. These are not only high in fiber, but also very filling and naturally low in fat.

Grains with Sautéed Vegetables

Sauté onions, celery, water chestnuts, and red pepper in a small amount of margarine or reduced stock. Add this cooked mixture to prepared wild rice, barley, couscous, or kasha, along with your favorite seasonings.

◆

Make mashed potatoes with nonfat cream cheese or sour cream, skim milk, or broth, and little or no butter or margarine. For a change, add a small amount of grated sharp cheese and a dash of cayenne pepper and bake a second time for a fluffy, flavorful potato casserole.

DESSERTS

Be sure to offer at least one low-fat dessert, such as fruit cobbler or angel food cake with fruit toppings.

◆

Keep the servings of higher-fat desserts small, or let guests serve themselves. Offering second helpings is often better than oversized first helpings.

◆

Serve cappuccino or café latte with skim or low-fat milk, sprinkled with ground cinnamon or cocoa. For the sweet tooth, add small sugar wafers or biscotti for a light and low-fat dessert.

◆

Make pumpkin pie with evaporated skim milk and save up to 11 grams of fat per slice. To lower the fat even more, make the crust with graham crackers or vanilla cookie crumbs and serve with a light whipped cream topping or nonfat frozen yogurt. You can also whip evaporated skim milk for a light topping.

Nonfat Whipped Topping

Pour one can of evaporated skim milk into a stainless steel mixing bowl, and place bowl with the whisk attachment in the freezer for approximately 30 minutes. Whip the evaporated milk on high, adding approximately 1/4 to 1/2 cup of powdered sugar, until stiff peaks form. Serve immediately or, if necessary, hold in freezer for up to 10 minutes. This topping is not for use on warm desserts.

◆

Consider alternatives to regular fruit pies (those with two crusts) with at least 14 grams of fat per slice. Serve a pie with just a bottom crust at about 7 grams per slice; a fruit crisp at 5 grams of fat per serving; or baked apples or poached pears with a crumb topping at around 1 gram of fat per serving.

◆

Impress your guests with a beautiful low-fat trifle for dessert instead of traditional desserts that may be higher in fat.

Low-Fat Trifle

Layer the bottom of a glass serving bowl with angel food cake or fat-free pound cake cubes. Next add a layer of fresh (or frozen, thawed, and drained) fruit chunks, such as strawberries, bananas, raspberries, or mangoes. Spread a layer of low-fat pudding, such as vanilla or banana, or fat-free frozen yogurt or ice cream. Repeat these layers once or twice. The pudding version can be refrigerated, but the ice cream or yogurt version should be eaten quickly (which shouldn't be a problem!).

IF YOU ARE A GUEST

Plan ahead for special meals by eating low-fat meals for a few days before the big event.

◆

Drink a glass of water or juice or nibble on a few crackers with low-fat cheese or a piece of fruit before the event so you don't arrive famished.

◆

When you do arrive, check out the appetizers or buffet table, decide which look most tantalizing, and limit yourself to those. Maybe just a bite or two of each will do.

◆

After an hour of socializing and nibbling hors d'oeuvres or buffet items, sneak off to the bathroom and brush your teeth. You'll be less likely to eat more!

◆

If the party is a sit-down dinner, choose your foods wisely, based on the portions and the ways they were prepared. Remember that any food can fit into your eating pattern as long as you have moderate portions of higher-fat foods.

◆

Keep portions of desserts small and don't deny yourself if there is something you would really like to try. Often a taste is all you need to satisfy a craving or your curiosity.

Index